Two Angels: brave people brought the story of Essiac Tea to the World

By Barry Bryant

Their work has resulted in hundreds of thousands being saved from debilitating disease.

Introduction

There is an old saying, "Pioneers get arrows in their backs." As I learned of the amazing stories of Dr. Gary Glum of Los Angeles, and nurse Rene Caisse of Brace, Ontario, Canada, I couldn't help thinking back to this old saying.

Rene Caisse was never properly recognized for her original discovery of this herbal tea remedy among the Chippewa nation of Canada (Ojibwa tribe) and using it to selflessly serve her doctor's cancer-ridden patients. The Canadian medical authorities ignored her work for many years until eventually public pressure made them consider her work. Then the authorities sidelined her discovery after she died in 1957.

But along came Dr. Gary Glum to rescue and resurrect her discovery. Dr. Glum was a very successful chiropractor in Los Angeles. He heard about Essiac Tea and thoroughly researched it. Then he began a campaign in the USA to inform the public of this discovery. He wrote articles, made public appearances, made radio interviews, etc. As awareness of Essiac Tea spread, the US medical establishment reacted harshly. They attacked Dr. Glum. His career was destroyed as a result of his bravery in facing up against the medical establishment to release this information to the world.

Yes, they were pioneers. They got arrows in their backs. In Dr. Glum's case, he eventually, under great pressure, left the USA and took a contract with the government of China. The Chinese medical authorities were very interested in his work, and he worked for many years in China further studying and perfecting the use of Essiac Tea. Then he dropped out of sight, and I do not know what eventually happened to him.

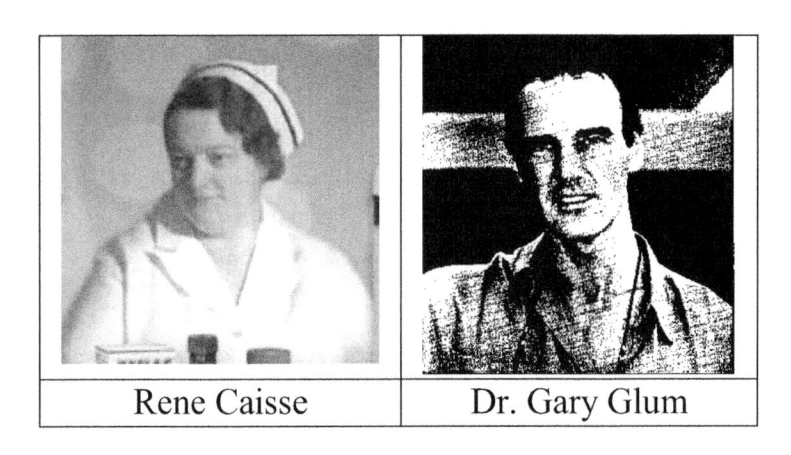

| Rene Caisse | Dr. Gary Glum |

So I have undertaken to write a book about all this. If you are new to alternative medicine and holistic healing, this information you will find interesting and important. If you are an old hand at all this, consider this a refresher course about Essiac Tea and how it can help you and your friends.

Dr. Gary Glum

Nurse Rene caisse had already passed way when Dr. Gary Glum began to investigate her work. He approached her family, offering the sum of $40,000 for access to her records. Thus he obtained the true formula for her Essiac Tea. Also obtained was a treasure trove of records and correspondence with further enriched his knowledge of her work.

When Rene Caisse reached retirement age, she had passed along her herbal formula to a Canadian company (the Respirin Corporation), with the belief that they would continue her work. But unfortunately, after Rene died, they shelved her project. Some say that this was a deliberate work to suppress her discovery, since an inexpensive natural herbal remedy was a threat to the pharmaceutical industry.

Anyway, knowledge of Essiac Tea would have died right there if Dr. Gary Glum had not come along. This is why I admire the man so much. Also, he freely shared the Essiac formula with the world. YEA!

Here is an interesting and widely read magazine article about him:

Interview with Dr. Glum (from Wildfire magazine, Vol. 6, No. 1)

Elisabeth Robinson: To begin with, Dr. Glum, can you tell us a little about how you became interested in the story you tell in Calling of an Angel, and how you learned about Rene Caisse and her work?

Dr. Gary Glum: A personal friend of mine knew this woman, whose name I have promised not to reveal, who was living in Detroit, Michigan. Twenty years ago she had been diagnosed with cervical cancer in a Detroit hospital where she was eventually given up as incurable and terminal. She was given about ten days to live.
 She convinced her husband to make a trip to Bracebridge, Canada where she went to see Rene Caisse. She was treated with the herbal remedy developed by Rene –Essiac – and in a short time she didn't have a cancer cell I her body. So after that time this woman began dedicating her life to disseminating information about Essiac in the United States. When I met her, she was the only person in possession of the original herbal formula who would relinquish it. I got the formula for Essiac from her.

That's how it began. When I started, all I had was a piece of paper. I thought what am I going to do with this? I decided the best way to go would be to find the information behind Essiac and put it in book form and bring it to the world.

I learned about Rene Caisse from Mary McPherson who was a very close personal friend of Rene's…not only a friend but also a patient. Mar's mother and her husband were also patients. They were all treated for cancer and cured by Rene.

Mary worked with Rene beginning in the 1930's and she had in her possession all these documents that had to do with Essiac over the 40 years Rene administered it. All the documents Rene had were destroyed by the Canadian Ministry of Health & Welfare at the time of her death in 1978. They burned all that information in fifty-five gallon drums behind her home.

Essiac is a non-toxic herbal cure for cancer that's been with us since 1922.

ER: Why?

GG: Because they don't want this information in the hands of the public or the press or anybody else. They indeed found out what Essiac was in 1937. The Royal Cancer Commission hearings had then come to the same conclusions that Rene had – that Essiac was a cure for cancer.

ER: What is Essiac exactly?

GG: Essiac is a non-toxic herbal cure for cancer that's been with us since 1922. It's a formula made from four very common herbs.

ER: I would guess that virtually every person in the U.S. today has been touched by cancer, either personally or through a loved one. If this information is true, and the effectiveness of this remedy is actually medically documented, many lives could be saved. Why do you think the information on Essiac is not more widely known?

GG: The information is withheld because cancer is the second largest revenue producing business in the world, net to the petrochemical business. Money and power suppress this truth.

No one has ever sought to sure [? should be cure] cancer – only to control it. I mean, the research institutes, federal governments, pharmaceutical companies, anybody that has a vested interest in the health care of cancer, including the American Cancer Society, the Canadian Cancer Society, any of these so-called benefactors to those who have contracted this disease – all of these institutions are involved in the money and power around cancer.

These institutions have influence over government and regulatory agencies such as the Food and Drug Administration. The FDA recommends only allopathic treatments for cancer and other life threatening diseases. It does not approve nor make legal alternative treatments of an kind.

ER: You're saying that Essiac is in a position similar to, for example, laetrile.

GG: Yes, the only reason laetrile was stopped – and it couldn't be stopped any other way – was through the insurance companies. The insurance companies sent down a directive to all allopathic physicians stating that they could not cover them in am malpractice suit in the event they were treating people with any substance not approved by the Food and Drug Administration.

ER: In your book you mention that the Brusch Clinic in Massachusetts worked with Rene Caisse and with Essiac, during the early 1960's. Is this clinic still doing research with Essiac.

GG: Dr. Charles A. Brusch is not practicing at this time. He was a personal physician to the late President John F. Kennedy. Dr. Brusch worked with Rene Caisse from 1959 to 1962. He worked with thousands of cancer patients. He also worked with the Presidential Cancer Commission, with others like Dr. Armand Hammer, the American Cancer Society, and the National Cancer Institute.

Dr. Brusch presented his findings after ten years of research. He had come to the conclusion that, in his own words, "Essiac is a cure for cancer, period. All studies done at laboratories in the United States and Canada support this conclusion."

Whereupon the federal government issued a gag order and said "You've got on of two choices, either you keep quiet about this or we'll haul you off to military prison and you'll never be heard of again." So we never heard another word out of him.

Brusch's Essiac patients included Ted Kennedy's son who had a sarcoma in his leg, and who had his leg amputated. He was being treated at the time by the Farber Cancer Institute in Boston, Massachusetts. Dr. Farber didn't know how to save him, because no one had ever lived with this type of sarcoma. So what he did was go to Dr. Brusch and say, how are we going to save Ted Kennedy's son? And Dr. Brusch made the suggestion to put him on Essiac, and after they did, he didn't have a cancer cell in his body. But all this information has been hidden from the general public.

ER: Why?

GG: Do you know wheather the remedy is being used or tested anywhere today in the U.S. or Canada?

GG: Right now Essiac is being used in every state in the United States, it's throughout Canada, into Mexico, it's in Australia, Europe, Asia, and recently, also in Africa. So the message of Essiac is beginning to make its way worldwide. But it's still known only on very limited basis.

Of course now you also have the problem of herbal distributing companies throughout the world that are substituting yellow dock and curly dock for sheep's sorrel, which is one of the critical ingredients in Essiac.

The sheep's sorrel is the herbal ingredient in Essiac that was found to be responsible for the destruction of cancer cells in the body, or their amalgamation where metastasized cancer cells actually return to the original tumor site.

That research was done by Dr. Chester Stock at Sloan-Kettering in New York for over a three-year period. But when they gathered that information, they withheld it from the general public – yet they gave it to the Canadian Ministry of Health & Welfare. The Canadian government then immediately banned that herb for sale and distribution.

ER: Banned a common weed like sheep's sorrel?

GG: Yes, sheep's sorrel is just a common weed that grows in abundance throughout North America and into Canada. Just a common weed. (Note: After this interview was completed, Wildfire learned from an herbalist in Canada that the Canadian government has recently banned St. John's Wort, also a common weed frequently used by herbalists)

ER: Well, it seems that banning sheep's sorrel would not be very effective if you could identify it for yourself.

GG: Yes, it's just a question of identifying the plant and then harvesting it correctly and drying it properly and then putting it together with the other herbs.
 Rene would harvest the sheep's sorrel – Rumex acetosella – when it was four to six inches high. She cut it back and it would grow up again, and she'd cut it back again. She would do that about three times and then she would let go to seed. It will grow to 14 to 18 inches.
    She would take the herb cuttings home and lay them out at room temperature to dry them. She'd let the cuttings sit there for three to four days before she'd begin turning the herbs. Then she'd turn them every two days until they were properly dried which took about ten days to tow weeks. It takes about a bushel of harvested sheep's sorrel to

produce on pound of the dried powdered herb which is used in the formula. (Note: As of March, 1993, Sheep Sorrel continues to be sold in Canada)

ER: Do you have the formula? It's not in you book. You do mention a video in the book.

GG: Yes, I have it. Anyone can get it from me, free of charge. We don't sell the video anymore. We simply mail the formula to anyone who asks for it.

ER: Sun Bear told me you had problems getting the book published and distributed. What kind of problems?

GG: There wasn't a publishing company that would publish it. No one wanted to run the risk of a wrongful death suit. So I published the book myself. And as soon as I did the IRS came in and slapped about a half million dollars in tax liens against me and said, "You know this has got nothing to do with taxes. It's all about cancer."

They actually started hauling the pallets of books out of my medical practice offices and confiscating them. I also had thousands of books that were confiscated by the Canadian government at customs. I have never received any of those books back. The only ones I have now are hidden in storage facilities.

ER: That's incredible – why do you think they are so interested in keeping this book out of circulation?

GG: Money and power, as I've said. Cancer is the largest revenue producing business in the world next to the petrochemical business. In Canada the book is being held up by the Ministry of Health & Welfare because they say it is "advertising."

ER: Advertising what? The video you don't sell any more?

GG: No, a cure for cancer.

ER: Can you explain what you mean by the publishers' fearing a wrongful death suit?

GG: What you're dealing with is giving people a formula that they can make and use in the privacy of their own homes without the approval of the AMA or FDA or anybody else. If any attorney or any family member should decide, for whatever reason, that the reason someone expired was from the use of Essiac, then you are putting yourself up for a wrongful death suit. The contention is that if it isn't approved by the Food and Drug Administration, there's no legality in using it when you're dealing with a life threatening disease.

When Rene Caisse set up her clinical trials in Canada to test Essiac, she was given government permission to treat terminally ill cancer patents who had been given up for hopeless by the medical profession. That was one criteria. Secondly, this was all to be certified by a pathology report. And third, she could not charge anything for her services. She agreed to all these criteria and proceeded to treat people with Essiac. Many she treated were still there 35 years later to bury her when she died at age 90.

The best that anyone can do is just try to disseminate this information to the public and let people make their own choices. That's all you can do. And just say, look, if you feel that Essiac has value in your life and the lives of your loved ones, you have the right to make this remedy and use it in the privacy of your own home and without anyone's approval.

You know, in 1937 Essiac came within three votes of being legalized as a treatment for cancer. People had garnered over fifty-five thousand signatures on a petition to allow Rene to continue to use Essiac. The only reason the vote fell short, she found out years later, was that the College of Physicians and Surgeons met and said to Parliament, if you don't respond to the political pressure and legalize Essiac, them we'll take a sincere look and give this woman a fair hearing. So Parliament didn't legalize Essiac.

So following the Royal Cancer Commission hearings, Rene was allowed to continue her practice but only within the criteria I mentioned before, which allowed the Ministry of Health & Welfare to restrict people's access to Essiac treatments.

I know this because I have a copy of the hearing transcripts which I got from Mary McPherson, which is some of the information that did not get burned when Rene died.

ER: You mentioned that earlier. What exactly was burned?

GG: All her research for that 40-year period of time. All the names, all her clinical data that she had collected. Her files and records.

ER: What about the records of the Brusch Clinic? It seems these would be convincing evidence.

GG: As far as I know all that material has been destroyed also. I knew that Rene had worked with Dr. Brusch from 1959 to 1962, so I went to Dr. Brusch's home in Cambridge, Massachusetts whereupon he delivered to me the only material he had let in his files on Essiac. One of those files was his own personal file where he had treated and cured his own cancer with Essiac. I have his personal records.

All the information in my book is verified by a sheet of paper with a signature and date on it, and those sheets and signatures are all originals. They are not copies.

ER: Have you had any personal experiences with Essiac?

GG: Yes, I can give you an example. He was a twelve-year-old boy named Toby Wood. He had acute lymphoblastic, which is one of the most virulent of all leukemia. He has been on chemotherapy for four years and radiation for three. His mother's only hope in life was to find a cure for him. She went everywhere. She tried every alternative treatment.

Her last stop was Dr. Alvazados in Athens, Greece where her son's white cell count was 186,000. He had no red blood cells and no platelets. He was hemorrhaging to death. So they transfused Toby in Greece and put him on a plane to Alaska where he was given less than five days to live.

I met his mother's sister in Los Angeles while I was putting the book together and she asked if there was any credibility here. We sat down and talked. She then borrowed the money for a flight to Anchorage, and delivered a bottle of Essiac. By the time she got there Toby was given three days to live. He was in a state of complete deterioration. He was given the Essiac and all the hemorrhaging stopped within 24 hours. Within three months all his blood tests were normal. I arrived in Alaska later that year and met him.

Toby Wood did die, and we finally found a pathologist who would do an exhaustive autopsy. We knew that he didn't have leukemia any more. We wanted to find out what was the cause of death. It took four months to get the report back. The pathologist autopsies the brain, testicles, and all life support organs, including the bone marrow. No blast cells were found in any life support organ. No blast cells were found in the bone marrow.   There were a few stray cells in the testicles and in the brain. Cause of death was damage to the myocardial sac of the heart, a result of the chemotherapy. This was the first report anywhere in medical history of anyone surviving lymphoblastic leukemia. That information was taken to AP and UPI but they said it was not newsworthy.

Our information on Essiac has been sent around the world twice through Publisher's Weekly magazine in a huge two-page ad. We received no responses at all from any publishing company worldwide, no producers, directors throughout the United States, no talk show programs, none of that. We can't access the media.

In fact we talked to Philip Scheffler, producer

of 60 Minutes. He read the book and we called him to ask whet her was going to do about it. He said nothing. I said, all the information in the book is verifiable. In other words, it's the truth. I said, if you're 60 Minutes why don't you expose me and Essiac as a fraud. He said, nope, can't do it.

We took it to Joe Donally who's the executive news producer for ABC in New York. We said why not give it to Peter Jennings, Geraldo Rivera, Ted Koppel, one of those. He said, nope. We asked why not. He said because his phone lines would be invaded with 65,000 phone calls. He went on to say he's got a mortgage on his house and he's looking toward retirement.

So that's the problem. No one wants this information disseminated. And it's not just the media, either. It includes the herbal companies who are now substituting the curly dock for sheep's sorrel. So people are getting the worn ingredients for Essiac, not to mention the five or six other formulas that are circulating which are different from the on I send out. These false formulas are being disseminated. There is a disinformation campaign going on here somehow.

ER: Has this disinformation campaign start just since your book has been out?

GG: Previous to my book, non of this information was available to the general public at all. The public had no information outside of a few assorted articles. Certainly the Essiac formula was not available to the general public at all. All that information was held by the Resperin Corporation in Toronto, Canada, which supposedly is a private institution.

However, they work hand and glove with the Canadian Ministry of Health & Welfare, who works directly with the American Food and Drug Administration and the National Cancer Institute in Bethesda, Maryland. The Essiac formula was never give to anyone by Resperin.

ER: Did the Resperin Corporation do any research on Essiac?

GG: They've done research since 1978 when the formula was relinquished to them by Rene for the purchase price of one dollar. As soon as they got the formula, they told Rene they head no further use for her. She had been under the distinct impression from the Ministry of Health & Welfare and the Resperin Corporation that she was to lead the research activities that thy so desperately wanted to put together.

But Rene had already done clinical trials. She had names and records. She thought the Resperin Corporation was politically powerful and had money enough to get Essiac into the public sector without compromising her values. The she found out the Corporation was working closely with the government and administration and the Ministry of Health & Welfare.

So now people who were terminally ill and given up as hopeless had to go through a federal bureaucratic maze to get the remedy. By then, for most of these people, it was too late. But even when people were cured that information was not released to the public.

Resperin ran research tests on Essiac. One test was conducted in Northern Canada and the documents were falsified. For example, on man was listed as dead who a few months later knocked on Rene's door and said, you know I want to thank you for the Essiac and being part of this experimental program. Yet he was listed as dead in the research project findings.

ER: It's beginning to seem amazing to me that any information at all about this remedy has survived the "conspiracy of silence" or outright destruction of records and so on.

GG: The only reason Essiac is known today is by word of mouth and because Essiac is what it is. What will keep Essiac known is its effectiveness. Rene said it years ago. She said, look, if Essiac doesn't have any merit let me put it out there. If it doesn't have merit, it will kill itself. Of course she knew full well if people had the correct hers, the remedy would stand on its own. And that's is exactly what Essiac has done over this period of time that we've been dissemination the information.

Rene also found that Essiac was a strong preventive. These finding were substantiated by Dr. Albert Schatz at Temple University who discovered the cure for tuberculosis.

Rene also found that Essiac would heal stomach ulcers within three or four weeks. She felt that ulcers were a precursor to cancer.

Sir Federick Banting, the co-discoverer of insulin, wanted to worked with Rene. She had clinical cases where a person on insulin discontinued it with the Essiac, since no one knew how Essiac would interact with the insulin. Apparently Essiac regulated the pancreas in cases of diabetes mellitus. So these people then became insulin free.

Another thing I've found with Essiac is that I've experienced almost perfect health. As you get older you think well, I'm forty now, these things happen. Well, these things don't have to happen. Since I've taken Essiac, I've experienced almost perfect health. It's amazing I sleep like a baby, have all kinds of energy, and no sickness, not even a cold or the flu.

I also worked with the AIDS Project Los

Angeles through their Long Beach and San Pedro districts. They had sent 179 patents home to die. They all had pneumocystis carinii and histoplasmosis. Their weight was down to about 100 pounds. Their T-4 cell counts were less than ten. The Project gave me five of these patients. I took them off the AZT and the DDI and put them on Essiac three times a day. Those are the only ones alive today. The other 17 are dead.

ER: That is incredible – but what kind of lives are they leading today?

GG: They're exercising three times a day, eating three meals a day. Their weight is back to normal. For all intents and purposes you wouldn't know they were sick a day in their lives. But this information is not being disseminated either, because AIDS project in Los Angeles makes over $100,000 a year.

Even the alternative health care professionals are out there to control not to cure. Alternative medical practice is jus a s mercenary and deceptive as the allopathic. No one wants a cure for cancer or AIDS.

Nationwide in the water we drink over 2,100 organic and inorganic chemicals have been identified, and 156 of them are pure carcinogens.

The alternative people are also in it for the money. What you're finding with Essiac is that it is not even allowed into the arenas of alternative health care. Do really what you've got out here is people continually perpetrating these lies against mankind. For money. For money and power. It's that simple.

Really once you think about it, the only reason we don't have solar power is that no one's figured out a easy to sell EXXON the sun. It's true. If they could, you'd have solar power. You know you'd have it.

ER: So, in your own personal experience, this herbal remedy works to – I'm going to just quote you here and say "cure" – cancer, thyroid conditions, diabetes, AIDS, ulcers…..

GG: It also cures the common cold. Essiac elevates the immune system. I've been taking one ounce a day for seven years, and in seven years I havens [? should be haven't] had a cold, flu or virus.

ER: And all of this from a simple native herbal remedy?

GG: Yes. Although Rene did alter it. She altered it with Turkish rhubarb root (Rheum palmatum). Turkish rhubarb has a 5,000 year history. It actually came up from India into China and then was taken by the British.

ER: Turkish rhubarb root certainly is not native in this country, nor available here. Herbals from foreign countries are fumigated and irradiated, so is it a food idea to use the Turkish rhubarb?

GG: You can substitute ordinary rhubarb root. The other two ingredients are burdock root (Arctium lappa) and the inner bark of slippery elm (Ulmus fulva). They are easy to obtain, usually. Sheep's sorrel, Rumex acetosella, is what destroys the cancer cells. The other three herbs are blood purifiers.
 Essiac elevates the enzyme system and gives all cancer patients and all AIDS patients the enzymes that have been destroyed. Essiac elevates the enzyme system; it elevates the hormone system, so the body can cure its own disease.

ER: What about quantities? Some herbals are toxic.

GG: Even its worst enemy could never lay claim that Essiac had any deleterious side effects whatever. ◆You can take Essiac safely, through all the clinical trial that have been done, up to six ounces a day. That's two ounces in the evening, two in the morning and two around noontime. That high dosage. Rene had the correct herbs and she used as little as one ounce a week.

But look at the difference between then and now. The food didn't have carcinogens in it, and neither did the water, nor the air. So what have we done? We've killed the air, killed the water, killed the food. So what's left?

Nationwide in the water we drink over 2,100 organic and inorganic chemicals have been identified, and 156 of them are pure carcinogens. Of those, if you have a tumor, 26 are tumor promoting, so they make the tumor larger. But of course this information is not available to the public either. Those figures are from tests conducted by the Environmental Protection Agency with have never been distributed to the public.

ER: How did you get the information?

GG: From a Ralph Nader organization out of Washington, D.C. The media has not disseminated this information. Another problem is that very few people read books any more. We can only hope they'll read Calling of an Angel. Of course, the problem right now is people getting the right herbs.

ER: Anything you'd like to add before we close this interview?

GG: I would like to say that I didn't do all this research because I feel I have a responsibility to myself. I know that I've done all I can to disseminate this information and bring it to the people.

I was the first person to release this information on Essiac, how to make it, to the general public and say, here it is, here's the formula here's the story. So now the story is out there and look what's happening – it's getting killed through a disinfromation campaign. I mean Harvard, Temple, Tufts, Northwestern University, Chicago –all these institutions have tested Essiac with the right stuff, and they all came to the same conclusions as Rene Caisse. But all that information has been buried.

ER: Gary, it's been very interesting to speak with you.

GG: It's been a pleasure. You're opening a Pandora's Box, you know, publishing this interview.

Nurse Rene Caisse

Rene Caisse was a nurse in Canada. In 1923 she observed that one of her doctor's patients, a woman with terminal cancer, made a complete recovery. Inquiring into the matter, Rene found that the woman had cured herself with an herbal remedy which was given to her by an Ojibway indian herbalist. Rene visited the medicine man, and he gladly and freely presented her with his tribe's formula. He explained that the Ojibway used their herbal remedy for both spiritual balance and body healing. The formula consisted of four common herbs. They were blended and cooked in a fashion which caused the concoction to have greater curative power than any of the four herbs themselves. The four herbs were Sheep Sorrel, Burdock Root, Slippery Elm Bark, and Rhubarb Root.

With her doctor's permission, Rene began to administer the herbal remedy to other terminal cancer patients who had been given up by the medical profession as incurable. Most recovered.

Rene then began to collect the herbs herself, prepare the remedy in her own kitchen, and to treat hundreds of cancer cases. She found that Essiac, as she named the herbal remedy, could not undo the effects of severe damage to the life support organs. In such cases, however, the pain of the illness was alleviated and the life of the patients was extended longer than predicted. In the other cases, where the life support organs had not been severely damaged, cure was complete, and the patients lived another 35 or 40 years. Some are still alive today.

Rene selflessly dedicated herself to helping these patients. She continued to treat hundreds of patients from her home. She did not charge for her services. Donations were her only income. They barely kept her above the poverty line. Over the years word of her work began to spread. The Canadian medical establishment did not take kindly to this nurse administering this remedy directly to anyone with cancer who requested her help. Thus began many years of harassment and persecution by the Canadian Ministry of Health and Welfare. Word of this struggle was carried throughout Canada by newspapers.

The newspaper coverage of Rene's work began to make her famous throughout Canada. Word was also spread by the families of those healed by Essiac. Eventually, the Royal Cancer Commission became interested in her work. They undertook to study Essiac.

In 1937 the Royal Cancer Commission conducted hearings about Essiac. Their conclusion was that Essiac was a cure for cancer.

Eventually the Canadian Parliament, prodded by the newspaper coverage and the widespread support generated for Rene by former patients and grateful families, voted in 1938 on legislation to legalize the use of Essiac. Fifty-five thousand signatures were collected on a petition presented to the Parliament. The vote was close, but Essiac failed by three votes to be approved as an officially sanctioned cure for cancer.

The complete story of Rene Caisse's life and struggles is told in a book written by Dr. Gary L. Glum entitled <u>The Calling of An Angel.</u> It tells of the documented recovery of thousands of cancer patients who had been certified in writing by their doctors as incurable. Rene continued her work for 40 years until her death in 1978. Rene had entrusted her formula to several friends, one of whom passed the formula along to Dr. Glum.

Of interest is that, in the 1960s, Rene Caisse worked with the well-known Brusch Clinic in Massachusetts. Dr. Charles A. Brusch was the personal physician for President John F. Kennedy. After 10 years of research about Essiac, Dr. Brusch made the following statement: "Essiac is a cure for cancer, period. All studies done at laboratories in the United States and Canada support this conclusion." A testimonial letter from Dr. Brusch is included in this handbook.

Further details of these interesting situations are explained in Dr. Glum's book. Instructions on how to order a copy of the book are contained in this handbook. Dr. Glum also distributes, free of charge, the complete formula for Essiac along with instructions on how to brew it. This information is also contained in this handbook. We are very indebted to Dr. Glum for his work.

About Essiac Tea

Rene Caisse's herbal formula contains four commonly occurring herbs:

Sheep Sorrel (Rumex acetosella).

The leaves of young Sheep Sorrel plants were popular as a cooking dressing and as an addition to salads in France several hundred years ago. Indians also use Sheep Sorrel leaves as a tasty seasoning for meat dishes. They also baked it into their bread. Thus it is both an herb and a food.

Sheep Sorrel belongs to the buckwheat family. Common names for Sheep Sorrel are field sorrel, red top sorrel, sour grass and dog eared sorrel. It should not be confused with Garden Sorrel. (Rumex acetosa).

Sheep Sorrel grows wild throughout most of the world. It seeks open pastures, rocky areas, and the shoulders of country roads. It is considered to be a common weed throughout the U. S. It thrives with little moisture, and is a good indicator of acidic soils.

The entire Sheep Sorrel plant may be harvested to be used in Essiac. Or just the leaves and stems may be harvested, and this allows the plants to be "reharvested" later. The plant portion of the Sheep Sorrel may be harvested throughout the spring, summer, and fall, to be taken early in the morning after the dew has evaporated, or late in the afternoon. Always harvest on a sunny day, as the plants need several days after a rain in which to dry properly. Harvest the leaves and stem before the flowers begin to form, since at this stage, all of the energy of the plant is in the leaves.

Roots may be harvested in the fall, when the energy of the plant is concentrated in the roots.

Never collect more than a year's supply of Sheep Sorrel, as it loses its potency when stored longer.

Burdock Root (Arctium lappa).

The roots, young stems, and seeds of the Burdock plant are edible. Young stalks are boiled to be eaten like asparagus. Raw stems and young leaves are eaten in salads. Parts of the Burdock plant are eaten in China, Hawaii, and among the Native American cultures on this continent. It is then, both an herb and a food.

The Burdock is a member of the thistle family. Remember the last time you cleaned cockle burrs from your clothing after a sojourn in the woods or meadow? Chances are, you had run up against this very friendly and helpful plant, you just didn't know it! It is a common pasture weed throughout North America. It prefers damp soils.

The first years the Burdock plant produces only green leafy growth. It is during the second year that it produces the long sturdy stems with annoying burrs.

The root of the Burdock plant is harvested. It is harvested from only the first year plants. The roots are about an inch wide, and up to three feet long. As with the Sheep Sorrel, the roots should only be harvested in the fall when the plant energy is concentrated in the roots.

Slippery Elm (Ulcus fulva).

The inner bark of the Slippery Elm tree has a long history of use as a food supplement and herbal remedy. Pioneers knew of it as a survival food. The powdered bark has long been used, and is still being used today, as a food additive and food extender, rich in vitamin and mineral content. Thus it also is a food.

The Slippery Elm is a favorite shade and ornamental tree. It is found throughout Canada and the United States. Only the inner bark of the Slippery Elm is used to make Essiac. Reliable supplies of Slippery Elm can be purchased in powdered form, and this is probably easier and preferable to harvesting it yourself. Should you wish to harvest your own Slippery Elm, strip the bark from branches, rather than from the main trunk system of the tree so that you do not damage the tree.

Turkey Rhubarb (Rheum palmatum).

We have all eaten Rhubarb. Its red, bittersweet stems are to be found in supermarket produce shelves each spring. We also eat rhubarb pie, jams and pudding. The Turkey Rhubarb is a member of the rhubarb family with roots, which contain a particularly strong and desirable potency.

The Turkey Rhubarb grows in China. The roots are harvested when the plants are at least six years old. This imported product has more potency than our native rhubarb. Rene Caisse began her Essiac work using the domestic rhubarb root, later discovering that the imported variety was more potent. However, most of the Turkey Rhubarb, which is now imported into this country is irradiated, which destroys many of its curative properties. So native rhubarb is now once again the rhubarb of choice for your Essiac blend. Rhubarb acts as a purgative.

Notes:

1. Should you choose to harvest your own plants, we strongly suggest that you follow the Native American practice of saying a short prayer to the plants before you harvest them. Thank them for the help they will give you. We believe that your plants, thus consecrated, will be more potent and effective.
2. Keep your eye out for classes on herbs and herb identification. Seek out herbalists who

are willing to educate you on plant identity, harvesting techniques, plant drying and processing.
3. Do not collect herbs from areas where insecticides or herbicides have been used. You want only organic herbs!

The Formula

Note: Many of you may prefer to purchase your Rene Caisse herbal drink in bottles. Others may wish to buy a package of the dried herb mixture and brew their own. We provide mail order instructions for both on page 14. The original formula, as given by Rene Caisse, is listed below. We are reprinting here her exact instructions for a two gallon batch, although you would probably not need such a large amount at one time. A smaller amount is offered in the mail order dried herbal package (see pg. 14) which makes 1/2 gallon of Essiac (which is a two week or four week supply, depending upon whether you take it once or twice daily).

Ingredients:

52 parts: Burdock Root (cut or dried) (parts by weight)

16 parts: Sheep Sorrel (powdered)

1 part: Turkey Rhubarb (powdered) or 2 parts domestic Rhubarb

4 parts: Slippery Elm (powdered)

This is the basic four herb formula which was presented to the Royal Cancer Commission in 1937 and was found by them to be "a cure for cancer". Later in her life, while working with Dr. Charles Brusch in Massachusetts, Rene added small potentizing amounts of four other herbs to her basic four herb formula. As provided to us by a woman who worked with Rene, and was given the formula by Rene, these extra four herbs were added as follows: Kelp (2 parts), Red Clover (1 part), Blessed Thistle (1 part), Watercress (0.4 parts). We consider the addition of these four extra herbs optional.

Supplies Needed:

4 gallon stainless steel pot with lid 3 gallon stainless steel pot with lid Stainless steel fine mesh double strainer, funnel & spatula 12 or more 16 oz. sterilized amber glass bottles with airtight caps, or suitable substitutes.

Preparation:

1. Mix dry ingredients thoroughly. Place herbs in a plastic bag and shake vigorously. Herbs are light sensitive; keep stored in a cool dark place.

2. Bring 2 gallons of sodium free distilled water to a rolling boil in the 4 gallon pot (with lid on). Should take approximately 30 minutes at sea level.

3. Stir in 1 cup of dry ingredients. Replace lid and continue to boil for 10 minutes.

4. Turn off stove. Scrape down the sides of the pot with the spatula and stir mixture thoroughly. Replace the lid.

5. Allow the pot to remain closed for 12 hours. Then turn the stove to the highest setting and heat to <u>almost</u> a boil (approximately 20 minutes). Do not let boil.

6. Turn off the stove. Strain the liquid into the 3 gallon pot. Clean the 4 gallon pot and strainer. Then strain the filtered liquid back into the 4 gallon pot.

7. Use the funnel to pour the hot liquid into sterilized bottles immediately, and tighten the caps. After the bottles have cooled, retighten the caps.

8. Refrigerate. Rene's herbal drink contains no preservative agents. If mold should develop, discard the bottle immediately.

Caution: All bottles and caps must be sterilized after use if you plan to reuse them for Essiac. Bottle caps must be washed and rinsed thoroughly, and may be cleaned with a 3% solution of <u>food grade</u> hydrogen peroxide (may be purchased in health food stores). To make a 3% solution, mix 1 ounce of 35% food grade hydrogen peroxide with 11 ounces of sodium free distilled water. Let soak for 5 minutes, rinse and dry. If food grade hydrogen peroxide is not available, use one half teaspoon of Clorox to one gallon of distilled water.

<u>Instructions for Use</u> (as reported by Dr. Glum)

1. Keep refrigerated.

2. Shake bottle well before using.

3. May be taken either cold from the bottle, or warmed (never microwave).

4. As a Preventative, daily take 4 tablespoons (2 ounces) at bedtime or on an empty stomach at least 2 hours after eating.

5. Cancer and AIDS sufferers, or other ill people, may wish to twice daily take 4 tablespoons (2 ounces), once in the morning, 5 minutes before eating, and once in the evening, at least 2 hours after eating.

Note:

> a. Stomach Cancer patients must dilute the herbal drink with an equal amount of sodium free distilled water.
> b. Many people have reported that Rene's drink works well to detoxify the body, and have taken it as a detoxification program.

Precaution: Some doctors advise against taking the herbal formula while pregnant.

Recommendation: Rene reported that the twelve hour brewing process is essential for Essiac to have its special powers. Essiac is being offered to the public in pills, teabags, and homeopathic drops. We do not recommend them. They may work, but they are not what Rene Caisse used, nor have we seen evidence that they work.

What It Does

The components of Rene's herbal drink interact to have an amazing effect on the human body. The chemicals, minerals, and vitamins all act synergistically together to produce a variety of healing agents.

<u>Sheep Sorrel</u>:

Sorrel plants have been a folk remedy for cancer for centuries both in Europe and America. Sheep Sorrel has been observed by researchers to break down tumors, and to alleviate some chronic conditions and degenerative diseases.

It contains high amounts of vitamins A and B complex, C, D, E, K, P and vitamin U. It is also rich in minerals, including calcium, chlorine, iron, magnesium, silicon, sodium, sulfur, and has trace amounts of copper, iodine, manganese and zinc. The combination of these vitamins and minerals nourishes all of the glands of the body. Sheep Sorrel also contains carotenoids and chlorophyll, citric, malic, oxalic, tannic and tartaric acids.

	Sheep Sorrel	

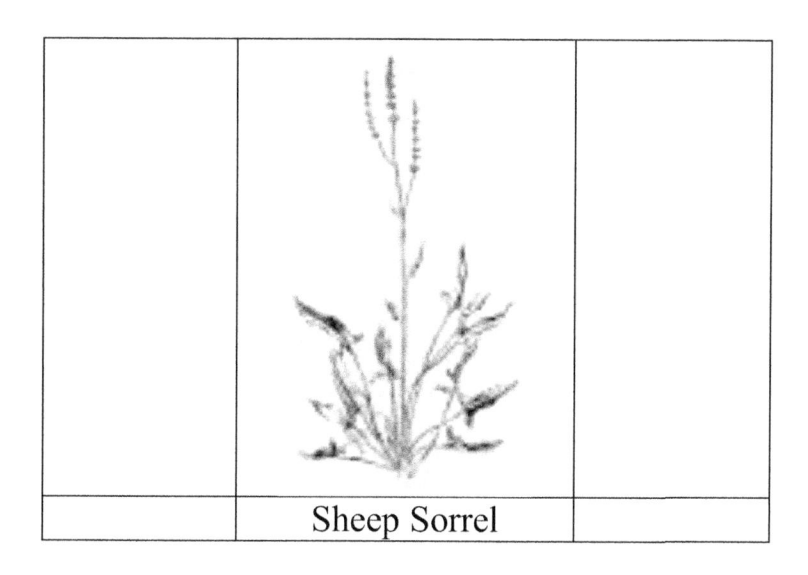

The chlorophyll carries oxygen throughout the bloodstream. Cancer cells do not live in the presence of oxygen. It also:

- reduces the damage of radiation burns
- increases resistance to X-rays
- improves the vascular system, heart function intestines, and lungs
- aids in the removal of foreign deposits from the walls of the blood vessels
- purifies the liver, stimulates the growth of new tissue
- reduces inflammation of the pancreas, stimulates the growth of new tissue
- raises the oxygen level of the tissue cells

Sheep Sorrel is the primary healing herb in Essiac.

Burdock Root

For centuries Burdock has been used throughout the world to cure illness and disease. The root of the Burdock is a powerful blood purifier. It clears congestion in respiratory, lymphatic, urinary and circulatory systems. It promotes the flow of bile, and eliminates excess fluid in the body. It stimulates the elimination of toxic wastes, relieves liver malfunctions, and improves digestion. The Chinese use Burdock Root as an aphrodisiac, tonic, and rejuvenator. It assists in removing infection from the urinary tract, the liver, and the gall bladder. It expels toxins through the skin and urine. It is good against arthritis, rheumatism, and sciatica.

Burdock Root contains vitamins A, B complex, C, E, and P. It contains high amounts of chromium, cobalt, iron, magnesium, phosphorus, potassium, silicon, and zinc, and lesser amounts of calcium, copper, manganese, and selenium.

Much of the Burdock Roots curative power is attributed to its principal ingredient of Unulin, which helps to strengthen vital organs, especially the liver, pancreas, and spleen.

	Burdock Root	

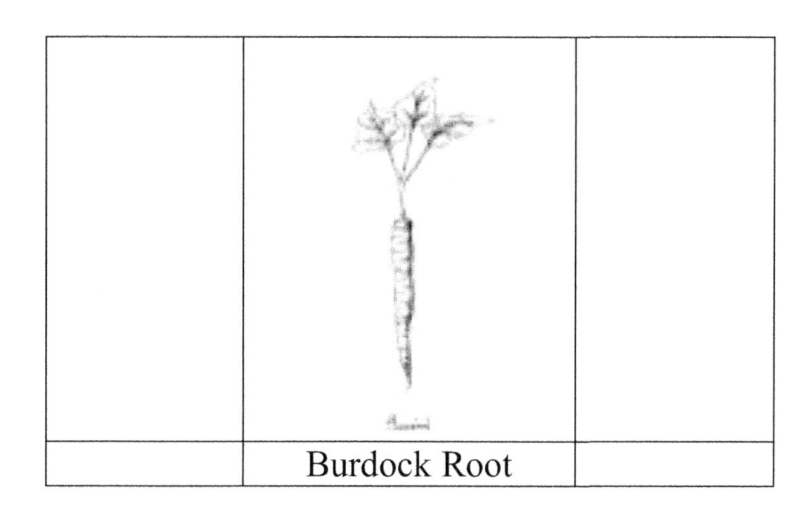

Slippery Elm Inner Bark

Slippery Elm Bark is widely known throughout the world as a herbal remedy. As a tonic it is known for its ability to sooth and strengthen the organs, tissues, and mucous membranes, especially the lungs and stomach. It promotes fast healing of cuts, burns, ulcers and wounds. It revitalizes the entire body.

| | Slippery Elm Bark Powder | |

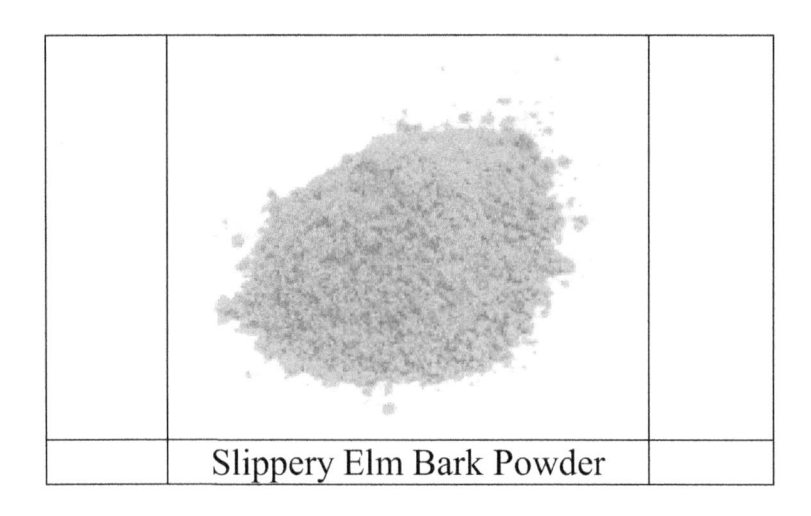

It contains, as its primary ingredient, a mucilage, as well as quantities of garlic acid, phenols, starches, sugars, the vitamins A, B complex, C, K, and P. It contains large amounts of calcium, magnesium, and sodium, as well as lesser amounts of chromium and selenium, and trace amounts of iron, phosphorous, silicon and zinc.

Slippery Elm Bark is known among herbalists for its ability to cleanse, heal, and strengthen the body.

Rhubarb

Rhubarb, also a well known herb, as been used worldwide since 220 BC as a medicine.

The Rhubarb root exerts a gentle laxative action by stimulating the secretion of bile into the intestines. It also stimulates the gall duct to expel toxic waste matter, thus purging the body of waste bile and food. As a result, the liver is cleansed, and chronic liver problems are relieved.

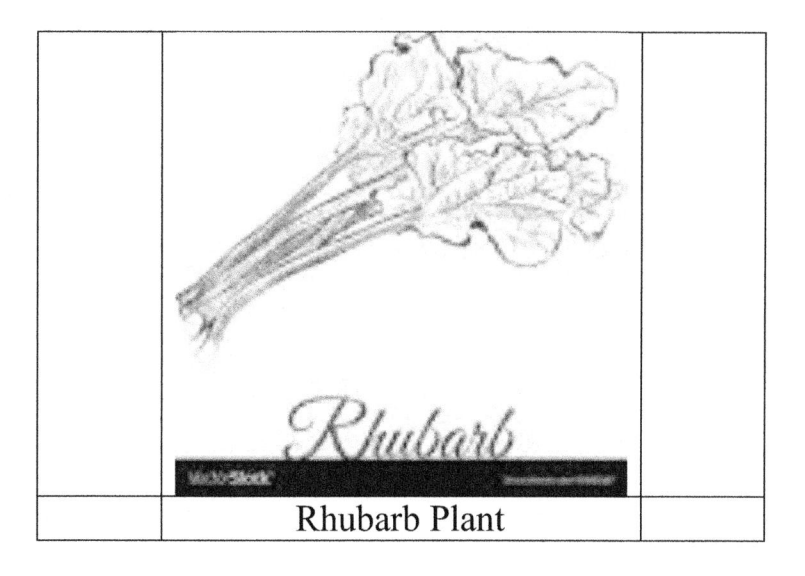

Rhubarb Plant

Rhubarb root contains vitamin A, many of the B complex, C, and P. Its high mineral content includes calcium, chlorine, copper, iodine, iron, magnesium, manganese, phosphorous, potassium, silicon, sodium, sulfur, and zinc.

Rene Caisse's Herbal Drink Has The Following Therapeutic Activity:

1. Prevents the buildup of excess fatty deposits in artery walls, heart, kidney and liver.

2. Regulates cholesterol levels by transforming sugar and fat into energy.

3. Destroys parasites in the digestive system and throughout the body.

4. Counteracts the effects of aluminum, lead and mercury poisoning.

5. Strengthens and tightens muscles, organs and tissues.

6. Makes bones, joints, ligaments, lungs, and membranes strong and flexible, less vulnerable to stress or stress injuries.

7. Nourishes and stimulates the brain and nervous system.

8. Promotes the absorption of fluids in the tissues.

9. Removes toxic accumulations in the fat, lymph, bone marrow, bladder, and alimentary canals.

10. Neutralizes acids, absorbs toxins in the bowel, and eliminates both.

11. Clears the respiratory channels by dissolving and expelling mucus.

12. Relieves the liver of its burden of detoxification by converting fatty toxins into water-soluble substances that can then be easily eliminated through the kidneys.

13. Assists the liver to produce lecithin, which forms part of the myelin sheath, a white fatty material that encloses nerve fibers.

14. Reduces, perhaps eliminates, heavy metal deposits in tissues (especially those surrounding the joints) to reduce inflammation and stiffness.

15. Improves the functions of the pancreas and spleen by increasing the effectiveness of insulin.

16. Purifies the blood.

17. Increases red cell production, and keeps them from rupturing.

18. Increases the body's ability to utilize oxygen by raising the oxygen level in the tissue cells.

19. Maintains the balance between potassium and sodium within the body so that the fluid inside and outside each cell is regulated: in this way, cells are nourished with nutrients and are also cleansed.

20. Converts calcium and potassium oxalates into a harmless form by making them solvent in the urine. Regulates the amount of oxalic acid delivered to the kidneys, thus reducing the risk of stone formation in the gall bladder, kidneys, or urinary tract.

21. Protects against toxins entering the brain.

22. Protects the body against radiation and X-rays.

23. Relieves pain, increases the appetite, and provides more energy along with a sense of well being.

24. Speeds up wound healing by regenerating the damaged area.

25. Increases the production of antibodies like lymphocytes and T-cells in the thymus gland, which is the defender of our immune system.

26. Inhibits and possibly destroys benign growths and tumors.

27. Protects the cells against free radicals.

Essiac and Chronic Fatigue, Lupus, Alzheimer's, Etc.

We have found Essiac to be very helpful to many people with Chronic Fatigue Syndrome, Lupus, Multiple Sclerosis, and Alzheimer's. To the best of our knowledge, all Lupus suffers who have taken Essiac have been significantly helped. We have also witnessed very rapid recoveries among chronic fatigue sufferers. Usually they report a very dramatic increase in energy. Some multiple sclerosis sufferers had less dramatic, but steady improvements in their conditions. One lady put her crutches away after taking Essiac for three months. Alzheimer's sufferers have reported improvements. Some with arthritis have reported improvement, although apparently not all arthritic sufferers are helped by Essiac.

It appears that Essiac's actions to remove heavy metals, detoxify the body, restore energy levels, and rebuild the immune system, all act to restore the body to a level to where it is able to better defeat the illness. In other words, Essiac rebuilds the immune system and improves the illness defeating ability of the body so that it can then rid itself of the illness.

Essiac and AIDS

In 1993 Dr. Gary Glum worked with an AIDS project in Los Angeles. The project had sent 179 AIDS patients home to die. They had pneumocystis carinii and histoplasmosis. Their weight was down and their cell counts were less than ten.

The project gave Dr. Glum five of these patients to work with. He took them off AZT and put them on a protocol of taking 2 ounces of Essiac three times a day. By February of 1994, all of the other patients had died. Dr. Glum's five patients were still alive. They were exercising, eating three meals a day, their weights were back to normal, and they had no appearance of illness.

An Endorsement by Dr. Julian Whitaker, M.D.

Dr. Julian Whitaker publishes a very informative and enlightening monthly newsletter named Health & Healing. It has 430,000 subscribers. In his November, 1995 issue he has an article titled "What I Would Do If I Had Cancer". He states that if he had cancer, he personally would follow a regimen which included changing his diet, taking the nutritional supplements Vitamin C, Shark Cartilage, Coenzyme Q1O, and he would take Essiac tea.

Dr. Whitaker has over twenty years of experience. He has written five major health books: *Reversing Heart Disease, Reversing Diabetes, Reversing Health Risks, A Guide to Natural Healing, and Is Heart Surgery Necessary?* Dr. Whitaker directs the Whitaker Wellness Institute in Newport Beach, California, which has treated thousands of patients. Should you desire information about subscribing to his newsletter, call (800)705-5559.

I highly recommend this newsletter to anyone who has a serious illness and wishes to become more knowledgeable about the complete range of healing modalities which are available. He also proscribes a 7 step 30 day wellness program "that will turn your life around".

Random Quotes From Rene Caisse:

"Though I worked each day from 9am to 9pm, my work was so absorbing there was no sense of fatigue. My waiting room was a place of happiness where people exchanged their experiences and shared their hope. After a few treatments, patients seemed to throw off their depression, fear, and distress. Their outlook became optimistic and as their pain decreased, they became happy and talkative."

"I could see the changes in some of the patients. A number of them, presented to me by their doctors after everything known to medical science had been tried and failed, being literally carried into my clinic for their first treatment. To later see these same people walk in on their own, after only five or six treatments, more than repaid me for all of my endeavors. I have helped thousands of such people. Some weeks I would have five or six hundred patients. I offered the treatment at no charge."

"Most importantly, and this was verified in animal tests conducted at the Brusch Medical Center and other laboratories, it was discovered that one of the most dramatic effects of taking this remedy was its affinity for drawing all of the cancer cells, which had spread, back to the original site at which point the tumor would first harden, then later soften until it vanished altogether. In other cases, the tumor would decrease in size to where it could be surgically removed with minimal complications. "

Disclaimer:

We are not permitted, nor do we, in this handbook make any claims that Rene Caisse's herbal formula will cure any disease. We have only gathered together in this easy-to-read handbook all of the already published information that is available to the general public about Rene's herbal remedy so that you may better make informed decisions. The documents which were used to compile this handbook are listed in the bibliography. Consult your physician before using Rene Caisse's herbal remedy. Copyright 1993 by James Percival. Publishing rights assigned to Bernard Barbieux Associates, Les Tres Peyres, Monbahus, France.

Bibliography & Reading List

The Calling of an Angel by Dr. Gary Glum, 1988, Silent Walker Publishing, PO Box 80098, Los Angeles CA, 90080 Tel: (310) 271 9931

The Essence of Essiac by Sheila Snow, 1993

Essiac: Nature's Cure For Cancer: An Interview with Dr. Gary Glum by Elisabeth Robinson, "Wildfire Magazine", Vol. 6, No. 1

Cancer Therapy by Ralph W. Moss, Ph.D., Equinox Press, 331 W. 57th St., Suite 268, New York, NY 10019, 1992

<u>Health & Healing</u> newsletter by Dr. Julian Whitaker, Phillips Publishing, 7811 Montrose Rd., Potomac MD 20854

My Favorite Source to Purchase Essiac Tea:

I purchase my Essiac tea from the following company in the United States. They give me courteous attention when I telephone them, their Essiac tea is made from organic herbs of the highest quality, their service is good, and their prices are fair.

I especially like that they make their liquid tea using structured water, the water developed by Dr. Masaru Emoto (he called it Hado Water). It is also a powerful healing agent.

Essiac can be purchased from:

Natural Heritage Enterprises
www.remedies.net

Tel: 888-568-3036

Their Products and Prices:

1. Bottles of Rene Caisse's Herbal Remedy: Bottles of the herbal remedy can be purchased by mail order for US$14.50 per 16 oz.

bottle. Made using only organic herbs, with rigid adherence to Rene's formula (her basic 4 herb formula enhanced with the additional 4 potentizing herbs).

2. **Dried Herbal Mix:** Should you wish to prepare your own Rene Caisse herbal drink, you may mail order packets of the dried herb combination. Each packet will allow you to prepare approximately one half gallon of the drink. The cost is US$12.00 per packet.

Letter from Dr. Charles Brusch:

Charles A. Brusch, M.D.
15 Grozier RD.
Cambridge, Massachusetts 02138

April 6, 1990

TO WHOM IT MAY CONCERN:

Many years have gone by since I first experienced the use of ESSIAC with my patients who were suffering from many varied forms of Cancer.

I personally monitored the use of this old therapy along with Rene Caisse R.N. whose many successes were widely reported. Rene worked with me at my medical clinic in Cambridge, Massachusetts and where, under the supervision of my many medical doctors on staff, she proceeded with a series of treatments on terminal Cancer patients andlaboratory mice and together we refined and perfected her formula.

On mice it has been shown to cause a decided recession of the mass and a definite change in cell formation.

Clinically, on patients suffering from pathologically proven Cancer, it reduces pain and causes a recession in the growth. Patients gained weight and showed a great improvement in their general health. Their elimination improved considerably and their appetite became whetted.

Remarkably beneficial results were obtained even an those cases at the "end of the road" where it proved to prolong life and the "quality" of that life.

In some cases, if the tumor didn't disappear, it could be surgically removed after ESSIAC with less risk of mestastases resulting in new outbreaks.

Hemorrhage has been rapidly brought under control in many difficult cases, open lesions of lip and breast responded to treatment, and patients with Cancer of the stomach have returned to normal activity among many other remembered cases. Also,intestinal burns from radiation were healed and damage replaced, and it was found to greatly improve whatever the condition.

All these patient cases were diagnosed by reputable physicians and surgeons.

I do knew that I have witnessed in my clinic and knew of many other cases where ESSIAC was the therapy used, a treatment which brings about restoration through destroying the tumor tissue and improving the mental outlook which reestablishes physiological function.

I endorse this therapy even today for I have in fact cured my own Cancer, the original site of which was the lower bowel, through ESSIAC alone.

My last Pete examination, where I Aces expedited throughout the intestinal tract while hospitalized (August, 1989) for a hernia problem, no sign of malignancy was found.

Medical documents validate this.

I have taken ESSIAC every day since my diagnosis (1984) and my recent examination has given me a clear bill of health.

I remained a partner with Rene repose until her death in 1978 and was the only person who had her complete trust and to whom she confided her knowledge and "know-howl of what she named 'ESSIAC."

Others have imitated, but a minor success rate should never be accented when the true therapy available.

Executed as a legal document.

Charles A. Brusch, MD

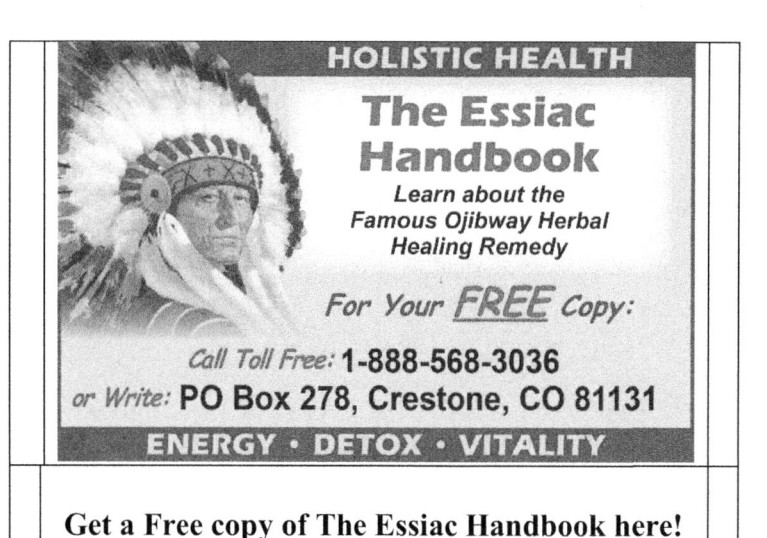

Get a Free copy of The Essiac Handbook here!

Printed in Great Britain
by Amazon